<u>My</u>
<u>Blood Pressure</u>
<u>Chart</u>

<u>Name</u>_____

<u>Date Started</u>_____

<u>Date Ended</u>_____

<u>By Catherine Coulter</u>

Fill out the charts to keep a record of your blood pressure. You can place a note each day as to how you felt or keep track of what you ate. It is portable enough to carry with you as you move about your day and to take with you when you visit your doctor.

For example:

Date: February 11, 2014

Time	Top Number (systolic)	Bottom Number (Diastolic)	Emotions
8 am	119	78	happy
1 pm	120	80	worried
9 pm	120	81	tired

Notes Today were a good day though I worried a little about my dog. I ate cereal, a sandwich, 2 apples, broccoli and a hamburger today

Date

Time	Top Number (systolic)	Bottom Number (Diastolic)	Emotions

Notes

Date

Time	Top Number (systolic)	Bottom Number (Diastolic)	Emotions

Notes

Date

Time	Top Number (systolic)	Bottom Number (Diastolic)	Emotions

Notes

Date

Time	Top Number (systolic)	Bottom Number (Diastolic)	Emotions

Notes

Date

Time	Top Number (systolic)	Bottom Number (Diastolic)	Emotions

Notes

Date

Time	Top Number (systolic)	Bottom Number (Diastolic)	Emotions

Notes

Date

Time	Top Number (systolic)	Bottom Number (Diastolic)	Emotions

Notes

Date

Time	Top Number (systolic)	Bottom Number (Diastolic)	Emotions

Notes

Date

Time	Top Number (systolic)	Bottom Number (Diastolic)	Emotions

Notes

Date

Time	Top Number (systolic)	Bottom Number (Diastolic)	Emotions

Notes

Date

Time	Top Number (systolic)	Bottom Number (Diastolic)	Emotions

Notes

Date

Time	Top Number (systolic)	Bottom Number (Diastolic)	Emotions

Notes

Date

Time	Top Number (systolic)	Bottom Number (Diastolic)	Emotions

Notes

Date

Time	Top Number (systolic)	Bottom Number (Diastolic)	Emotions

Notes

Date

Time	Top Number (systolic)	Bottom Number (Diastolic)	Emotions

Notes

Date

Time	Top Number (systolic)	Bottom Number (Diastolic)	Emotions

Notes

Date

Time	Top Number (systolic)	Bottom Number (Diastolic)	Emotions

Notes

Date

Time	Top Number (systolic)	Bottom Number (Diastolic)	Emotions

Notes

Date

Time	Top Number (systolic)	Bottom Number (Diastolic)	Emotions

Notes

Date

Time	Top Number (systolic)	Bottom Number (Diastolic)	Emotions

Notes

Date

Time	Top Number (systolic)	Bottom Number (Diastolic)	Emotions

Notes

Date

Time	Top Number (systolic)	Bottom Number (Diastolic)	Emotions

Notes

Date

Time	Top Number (systolic)	Bottom Number (Diastolic)	Emotions

Notes

Date

Time	Top Number (systolic)	Bottom Number (Diastolic)	Emotions

Notes

Date

Time	Top Number (systolic)	Bottom Number (Diastolic)	Emotions

Notes

Date

Time	Top Number (systolic)	Bottom Number (Diastolic)	Emotions

Notes

Date

Time	Top Number (systolic)	Bottom Number (Diastolic)	Emotions

Notes

Date

Time	Top Number (systolic)	Bottom Number (Diastolic)	Emotions

Notes

Date

Time	Top Number (systolic)	Bottom Number (Diastolic)	Emotions

Notes

Date

Time	Top Number (systolic)	Bottom Number (Diastolic)	Emotions

Notes

Date

Time	Top Number (systolic)	Bottom Number (Diastolic)	Emotions

Notes

Date

Time	Top Number (systolic)	Bottom Number (Diastolic)	Emotions

Notes

Date

Time	Top Number (systolic)	Bottom Number (Diastolic)	Emotions

Notes

Date

Time	Top Number (systolic)	Bottom Number (Diastolic)	Emotions

Notes

Date

Time	Top Number (systolic)	Bottom Number (Diastolic)	Emotions

Notes

Date

Time	Top Number (systolic)	Bottom Number (Diastolic)	Emotions

Notes

Date

Time	Top Number (systolic)	Bottom Number (Diastolic)	Emotions

Notes

Date

Time	Top Number (systolic)	Bottom Number (Diastolic)	Emotions

Notes

Date

Time	Top Number (systolic)	Bottom Number (Diastolic)	Emotions

Notes

Date

Time	Top Number (systolic)	Bottom Number (Diastolic)	Emotions

Notes

Date

Time	Top Number (systolic)	Bottom Number (Diastolic)	Emotions

Notes

Date

Time	Top Number (systolic)	Bottom Number (Diastolic)	Emotions

Notes

Date

Time	Top Number (systolic)	Bottom Number (Diastolic)	Emotions

Notes

Date

Time	Top Number (systolic)	Bottom Number (Diastolic)	Emotions

Notes

Date

Time	Top Number (systolic)	Bottom Number (Diastolic)	Emotions

Notes

Date

Time	Top Number (systolic)	Bottom Number (Diastolic)	Emotions

Notes

Date

Time	Top Number (systolic)	Bottom Number (Diastolic)	Emotions

Notes

Date

Time	Top Number (systolic)	Bottom Number (Diastolic)	Emotions

Notes

Date

Time	Top Number (systolic)	Bottom Number (Diastolic)	Emotions

Notes

Date

Time	Top Number (systolic)	Bottom Number (Diastolic)	Emotions

Notes

Date

Time	Top Number (systolic)	Bottom Number (Diastolic)	Emotions

Notes

Date

Time	Top Number (systolic)	Bottom Number (Diastolic)	Emotions

Notes

Date

Time	Top Number (systolic)	Bottom Number (Diastolic)	Emotions

Notes

Date

Time	Top Number (systolic)	Bottom Number (Diastolic)	Emotions

Notes

Date

Time	Top Number (systolic)	Bottom Number (Diastolic)	Emotions

Notes

Date

Time	Top Number (systolic)	Bottom Number (Diastolic)	Emotions

Notes

Date

Time	Top Number (systolic)	Bottom Number (Diastolic)	Emotions

Notes

Date

Time	Top Number (systolic)	Bottom Number (Diastolic)	Emotions

Notes

Date

Time	Top Number (systolic)	Bottom Number (Diastolic)	Emotions

Notes

Date

Time	Top Number (systolic)	Bottom Number (Diastolic)	Emotions

Notes

Date

Time	Top Number (systolic)	Bottom Number (Diastolic)	Emotions

Notes

Date

Time	Top Number (systolic)	Bottom Number (Diastolic)	Emotions

Notes

Date

Time	Top Number (systolic)	Bottom Number (Diastolic)	Emotions

Notes